Food and Nutrition Workbook for Children

for parents and teachers too

Michael R. Basso

I0417585

Edited by Dorothy Scarfone

First Edition

Copyright © 2011 by Michael R. Basso
ISBN: 978-1456379926

About the Author

Michael has written and co-authored a variety of children's books designed to build tolerance, respect and wellness. Michael has written more than 150 popular articles on wellness and holistic health. Dr. Basso has also written for the Yale Journal for the Humanities in Medicine as well as professional articles in Psychiatry and Neuroscience.

Michael R. Basso has significant experience as a leader in quality and reliability engineering and management in industry, as well as being a college level educator in psychology at Yale University and the University of Connecticut. His experience also includes being a consultant, researcher, and newspaper columnist. Michael is the president of the Connecticut Holistic Health Association.

Dr. Basso has a Ph.D. in professional psychology and biomedical systems, an MS in engineering science, and an MBA with a focus in executive leadership and an interdisciplinary Professional Development Diploma in pathophysiology, neural systems, and education. He also holds a BS in electrical engineering. Michael is certified in quality and reliability engineering and quality auditing, as well as variety of health related areas

Preface – for parents and teachers too

Food and nutrition are among the most important things to consider in your life - regardless of if you are well or not so well. Every aspect of our body and mind are influenced by food, from the time our bodies are forming before we are born and throughout our lives.

Good nutrition influences our grades in school, how we perform in sports and even how we get along with others. In this workbook, essential nutrients will be discussed along with the influence of not so good foods, fad diets and more. We will consider cultural and religious aspects of food and eating that may be encountered in school.

The purpose of this little book is to provide some general ideas and tips in the form of a story – not to suggest a diet, as everyone is different and no one diet works for everyone and in fact some diets can be harmful to some people.

Questions will be included in the workbook section to reinforce the materials learned.

Please be advised that this book is not meant for the diagnosis and/or treatment of any disease. Parents or guardians are advised to consider seeking the advice of an expert whom they trust and feel safe with.

"Dad, why do we have to eat? It is soooo much a waste of time – except maybe eating ice cream and chips. They make us happy, so they are not so much as waste of time."

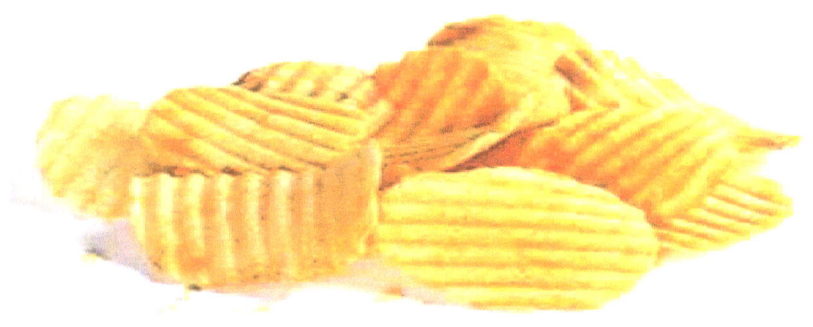

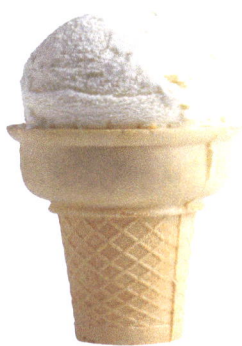

"Darling, we need to eat to live."

"Huh."

"Yes, Priscilla, your dad is right."

"Oh, Gosh, mom. Please don't make this into a lecture. We had enough of that in school. They said that sweets were making us sick, so they took all of the candy out of the vending machines. It was awful, mom. I don't even want to think about it."

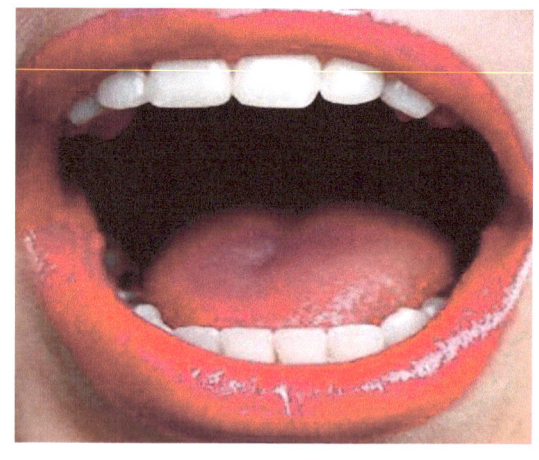

"They even told us to chew carefully, like we were in kindergarten – what's the difference how we chew?"

"Come on, you know that digestion starts with chewing in the mouth, then it continues in the stomach and on into the 3 parts of the small intestine and then the 3 parts of the large intestine."

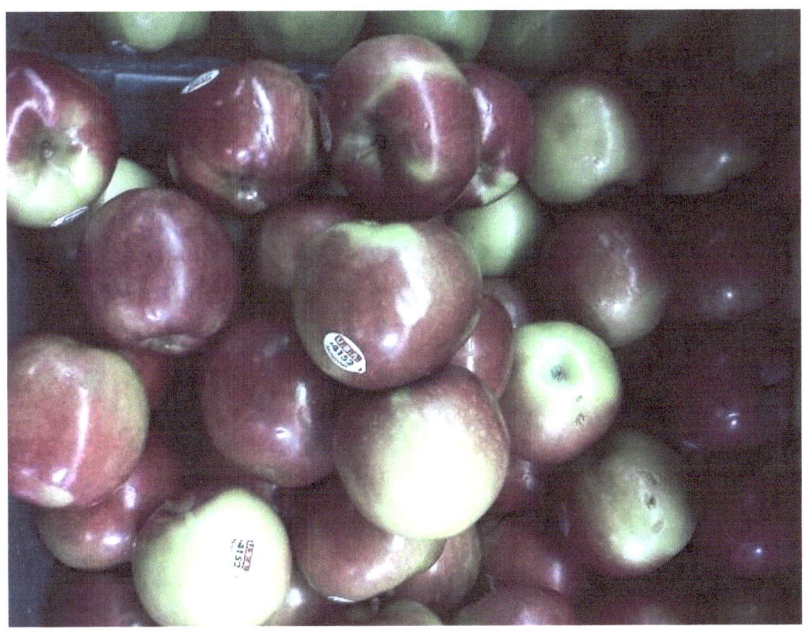

"I guess I will review my biology books to remind me of the details – thanks for the reminder, now it is becoming interesting!"

"Poor baby!"

"Why did they do it with the sweets, mom?"

"Well, honey, there are many good reasons that the junk food is gone – obesity, diabetes, even panic attacks can be caused by sweets."

[young boy]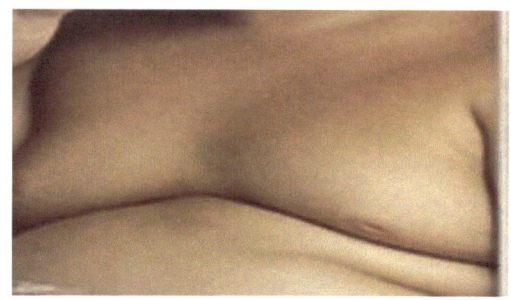

"The fat stuff and diabetes thing has been drummed into our heads, but what the heck are you talking about with the panic attack stuff, mom?"

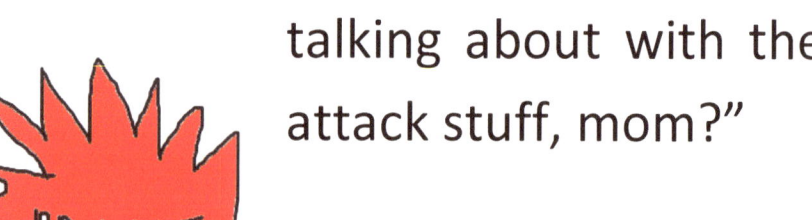

"First of all, your brain and nervous system uses most of the glucose - sugar – that our bodies get from our foods. In order for our brains to use the glucose, there must be

- Oxygen from well functioning lungs

- Vitamins, minerals, fats and water from healthy digestive systems

- All that stuff taken to the brain and nervous system by a healthy heart and cardiovascular system

- Waste is   eliminated by healthy livers, intestines, kidneys and even our lungs and skin.

"Ok, Ok, what's that have to do with panic attacks?"

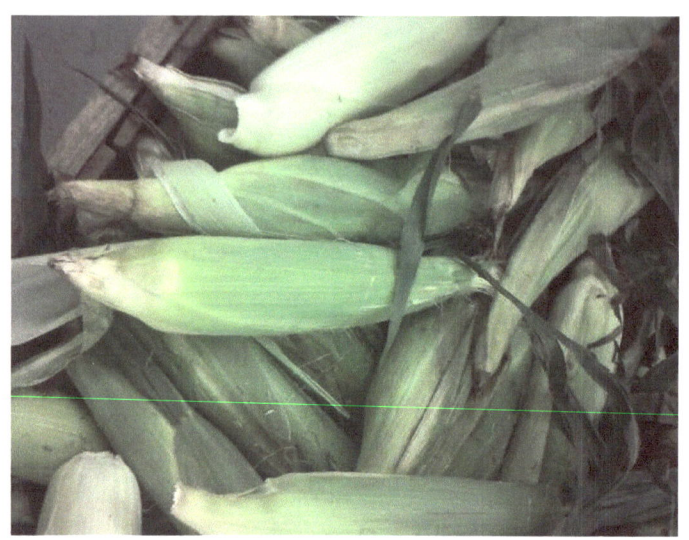

"When you eat too many sweets or drink it, your body gets full of sugar, so it has to get rid of and/or store the excess somehow. That high fructose corn syrup is just another type of sugar and it's everywhere – even in the soda that you think is good for you; it's not. You body has to deal with the excess."

"I don't get it, mom. I thought corn was good for you."

"High fructose corn syrup is a kind of sugar processed from corn – it's real sweet too and it's very different from whole corn – even that is on the sweet side so please do not overdo it. Same with bananas, oranges and lots of other sweetish foods."

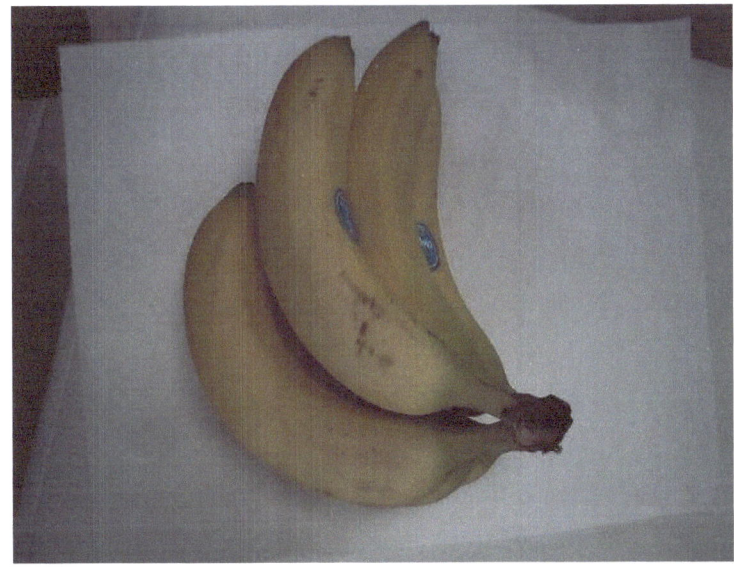

"Anyway, weird as it may sound, sweets – even too much fruit in some cases, can make the pancreas send out lots of

in sul in

to move the sugar out of our blood. It can make us store sugar as fat or even make us pee a lot to get rid of it. Then sometimes the sugar in our blood, that helps our brains work, can get too low."

"When the sugar in the blood gets too low, some people -

Get panic attacks

Get real hyper and can't focus
or

Even get so tired that they can't pay attention in class, do their homework, or even play sports."

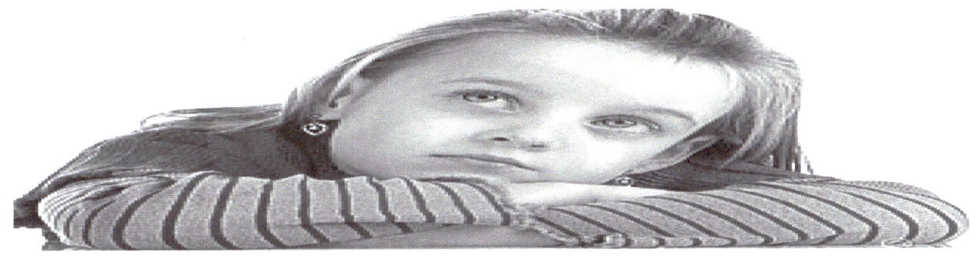

"Wow, our coach was just talking about kids who get too skinny – they sometimes get so tired when sports they are playing that they can't do anything. She even said that kids sometimes get violent when the sugar in their blood gets too low."

"She said that it is important to get the -

Right amount of exercise

Right amount of sleep

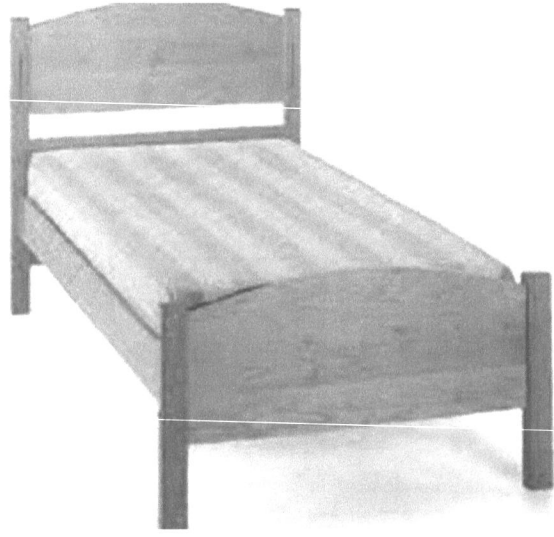

And the

Right amount of the right kind of food for us.

"She even said that in different kinds of weather that some people eat differently. The coach told us that water was food too – how weird."

"Water is very important and can make us very sick if we don't have enough –

We can get

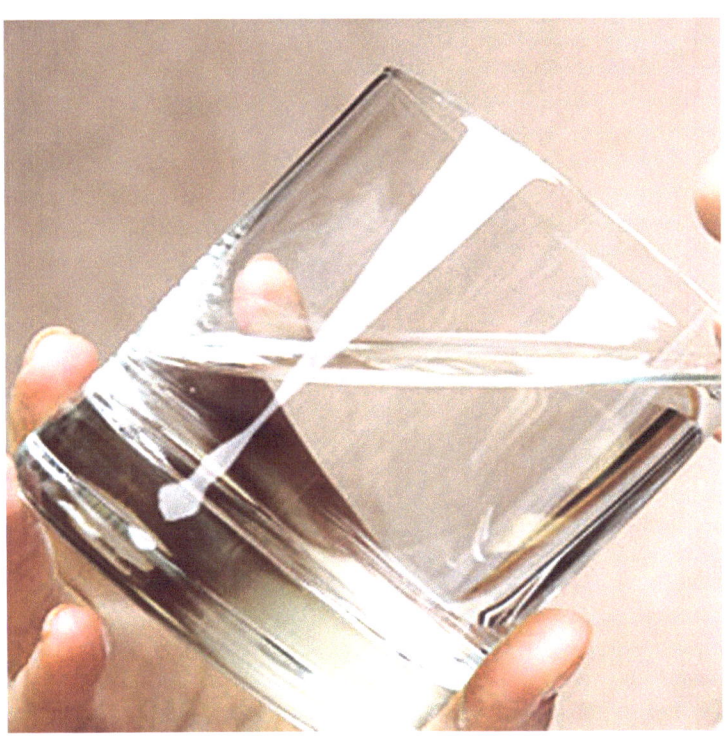

de hy drat ed."

"What does that mean?"

"Well, our bodies are more than 90 percent water – if you think about it. We need water to

Help digest food
Keep our skin healthy

Keep our brains healthy. We can even get bad headaches when we don't have enough water.

Some people don't think that as we lose weight that any medicines that someone might take – especially in hot weather – could get more concentrated!"

"Cool!"

"Mom, that Jewish kid in my class will only eat food that goes to church or something – what are they talking about?"

"Well, honey, some people will only eat Kosher foods – they are blessed by a Rabbi. Rabbis are like ministers or priests."

"That kid from California is on a special diet called

mac ro bi ot ics

what's that?"

"They believe that foods have a special something about them that is different from vitamins and that sort of stuff – they say that some foods are

YIN and other foods are YANG

And that you have to have the right amount of each or you will not be well.

They also think that you have to eat different foods during different seasons if you want be well."

"No matter what kind of diet you have, there are some guidelines to think about –

1) It's important to have foods that have the right amount of protein – protein helps us to grow and it makes our muscles be strong. We are vegetarians so we don't eat meat or eggs, and we get our protein from beans, peanut butter, almonds and some dairy. But we must be sure that we get enough vitamin B12 – so

we get that from some kinds of seaweed. We also know that too much

<u>Phos phor us</u>, from beans and grains is not so good either, so we read lots about that stuff too."

2)Carbohydrates give us energy. It's better if it comes from whole grains, like whole wheat pasta, whole grain oatmeal and some types

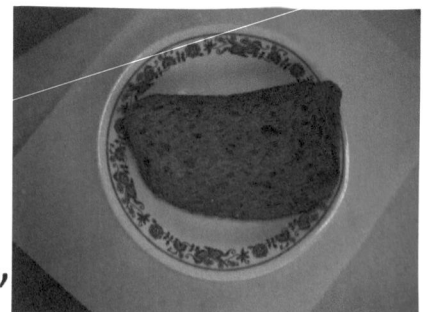

of whole wheat bread."

3)Vitamins are very important –

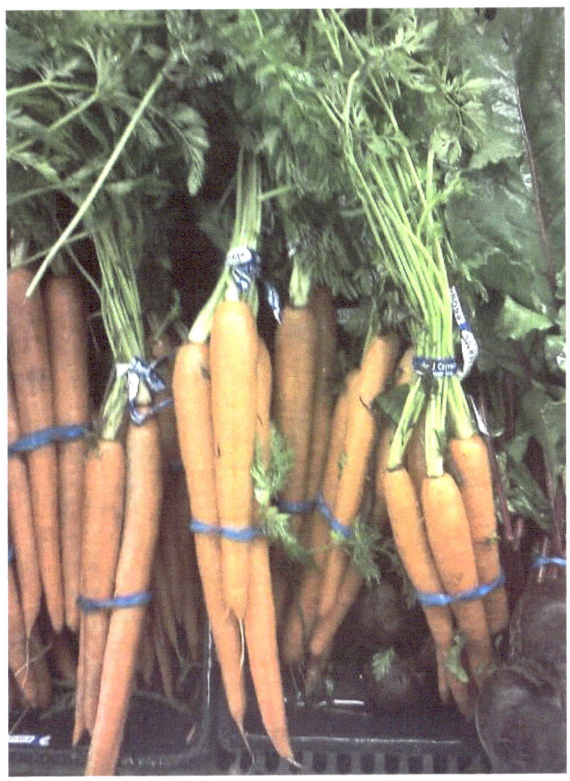

a. Vitamin A is good for our skin, our immune systems and lots of other things – we get it from

beta carotene in carrots, cantaloupes, and even parsley

b. The B vitamins are important to give us energy and even to make our nervous systems healthy. It is important to have the whole B complex (B1, B2, B3, B5, B6, B12...folic acid) or our body can go out of balance. Some people have trouble absorbing some of the B vitamins, so they take them under the tongue in a form that melts easily.

c. Vitamin C is very important for our immune systems too. Some people don't know that it makes our blood vessels and even our skin strong. Vitamin C works with something called bi o flav en oids — found in the white parts of oranges, peppers and even in parts of apples.

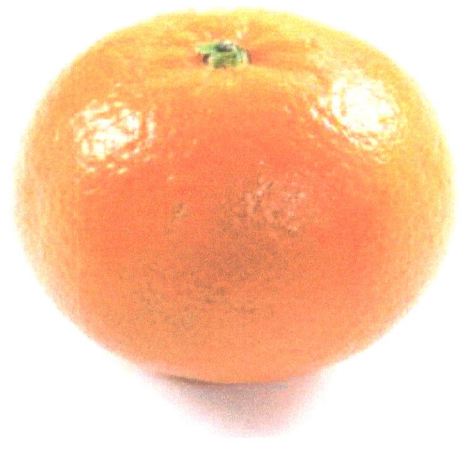

"Mom, is it true that Vitamin C works along with other things? They said in school that it works along with Iron, that bio stuff, something called magnesium too and that that magnesium stuff needs B6 to work properly and that that needs the rest of the B vitamins that Zinc was important too – huh complicated stuff."

"All that is true, Priscilla."

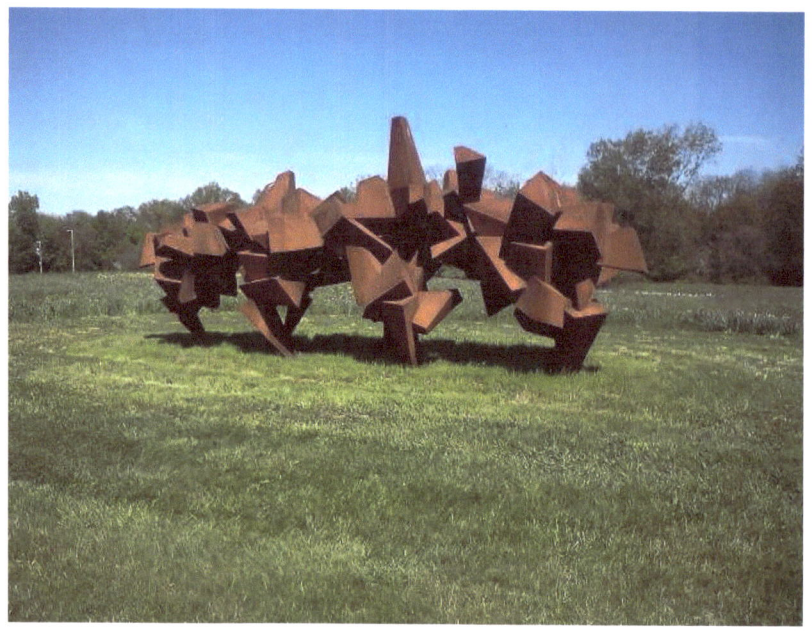

d. Vitamin E and other vitamins are also important to have healthy brains, skin and other parts of our bodies.

4) Minerals are important too.

a. For example, iron is needed to make our blood healthy, so it can bring oxygen to our brains to make us smart and have lots of energy. As girls mature, they may need even more iron than boys.

5) Fats, like the famous Omega 3 fatty acids are real inportant – they are learning more and more about how this stuff can make our moods better and even help with some kinds of depression.

"We are vegetarians, mom, how are we going to get that stuff. I saw on TV that it comes from fish."

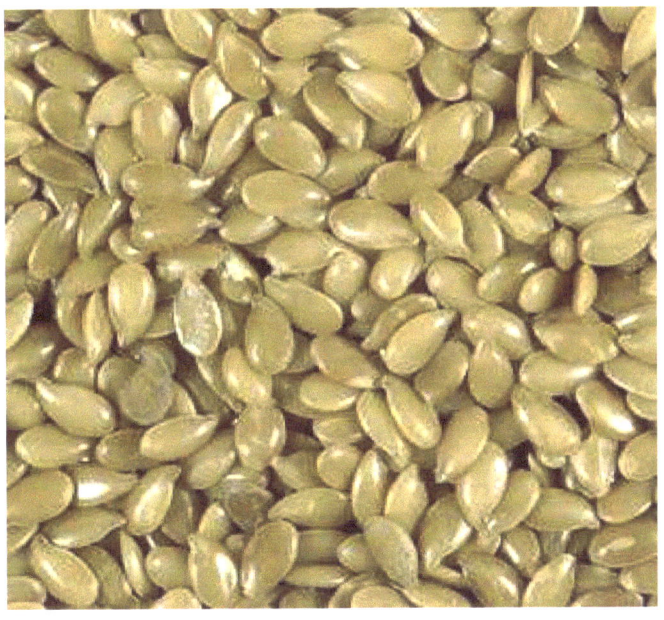

"Well,

sometimes the TV stuff is there because

somebody is trying to sell something. We can also get Omega 3 and other nutrients without meat, fish or eggs – for example Omega 3 can come from flax seeds and lots of other vegetable sources."

"Wow, I guess you have to know what you are doing to be smart about eating – being a vegetarian is more than not hurting animals or wasting energy by eating chips and   rice."

"Hey   at   least   eat
brown   whole
grain   rice!"

"Mom, this kid in school used to hear voices and was acting very weird – when he started eating better foods with lots of B – vitamins, foods high in zinc and magnesium and some other things - and not so much junk food; the voices went away and he starting doing very well in school again."

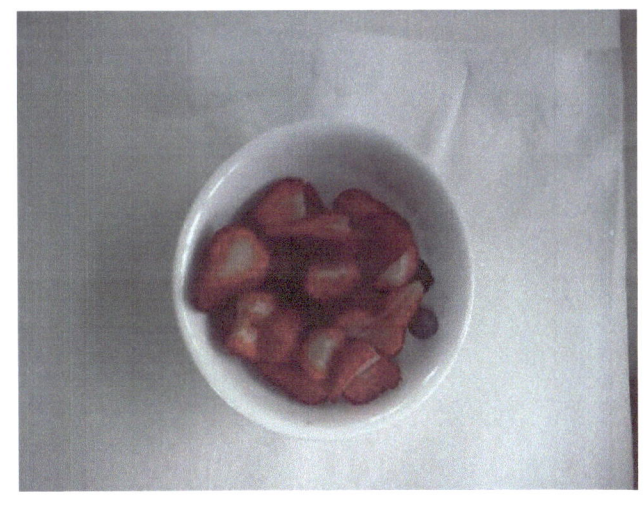

"Honey, we scientists are learning lots about how kids foods help who are sick and even to help kids do well in school. But please don't assume that food is always all these kids need who are very sick – like hearing voices."

"Some kids, especially those who may have had antibiotics for something, are also helped by

Pro bi to ics

They put back the

Good bacteria

That is naturally in our tummies, our mouths and other places. Some people like to add fresh fruit, such as berries."

"Wow that's cool mom – never thought about that."

"There are also different kinds of fiber – another thing to know about and not to tell others to do unless you speak to their parents. Some people are very sensitive to certain foods and too much of some types of fiber can actually make some matters worse – it can irritate their intestines."

"On the other hand honey, some kids with skin problems are helped by

>Drinking more water

>Having the right amount of the right type of fiber

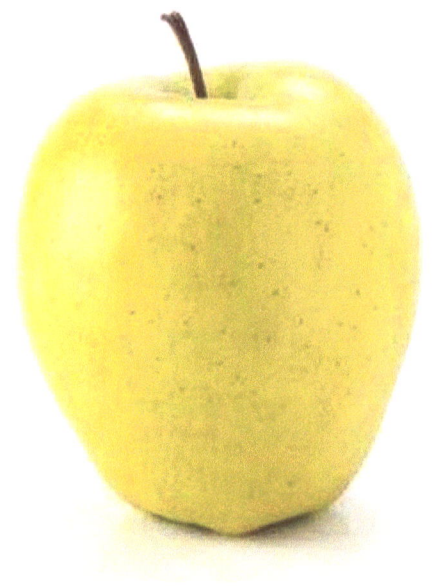

>Include probiotic foods in their diets

>Have the right amount of vitamins, minerals and fats in their foods as part of a balanced diet."

"It is very important that you talk to your parents about foods and other health related things –and please do not interfere with what other kids are doing, including taking medications."

"Ok, mom."

"Please keep in mind that some other foods, even good ones can cause problems. For example, some people are allergic to certain foods – like the

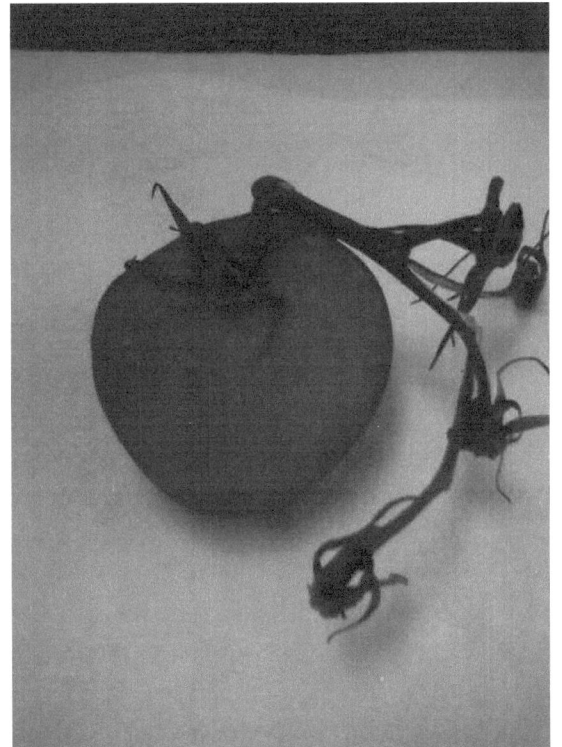

nightshades, which include tomatoes, potatoes, eggplant, green peppers and even tobacco."

"Huh."

"That right kiddo, please be careful what you suggest to other kids and please don't interfere with what kids parents want their kids to eat."

"Well, ma, that kid who is always sick. Well, my friend Jamie told her to eat more garlic because it is good for so many things."

"I am glad you told me

about that, Prissy."

"Why – what could possible be wrong with garlic the best of all foods?"

"Garlic is a great example! Some people are on medications that can make people bleed when it is mixed with garlic!"

"Oh, Gosh, mom!!! She was taking some kinda meds – I'll tell her. Wow they just told us a story about how some cows ate a

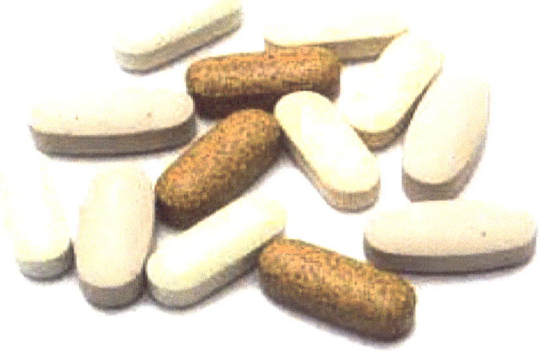

bunch of moldy red clover and bled to death."

"Please - I'll tell Mrs. Rosenblatt."

"We were also going to talk about supplements as she asked me about them at the PTA meeting."

"Are vitamins and other supplements good for us?"

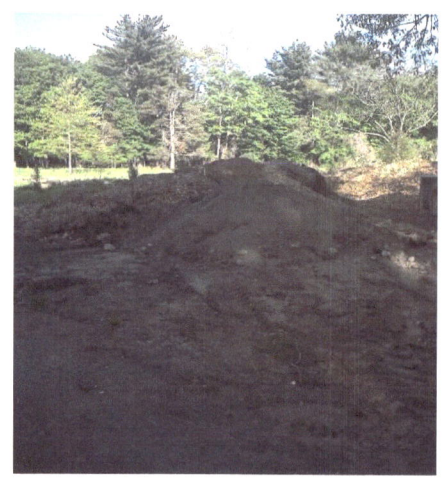

"While some 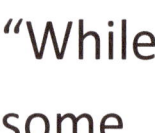 there may be advantages to supplements -

I prefer to get the nutrients from ripe foods that are grown on good soils."

"Come on, mom. Now you are getting out of control! – dirt is dirt. Who cares about the soils?"

"Well, there are different minerals in different soils in different parts of the world. Also, when we keep on growing stuff we deplete the soil."

I heard something about there are soils in parts of Japan not having enough iodine and the soils in parts of Egypt not having enough zinc on TV. They said that because of the depleted soil that the foods didn't have enough nutrients and then the foods can't make us healthy."

"Now – there is my well nourished and smart daughter."

"mom!"

Workbook Section

It is Ok for others to help us here & to look at other books, including our science books

Please share a few points to know about digestion, starting from the mouth

1)

2)

3)

4)

5)

6)

Please name some organs that are important to get food and oxygen to our brains

1)

2)

3)

4)

5)

Please let us know a few things about the B – Complex vitamins

1)

2)

3)

4)

5)

6)

Please tell us about food allergies, including something about the nightshades

1)

2)

3)

4)

5)

6)

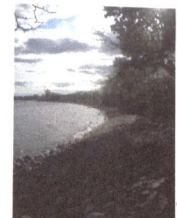 Why is water so important?

1)

2)

3)

4)

5)

6)

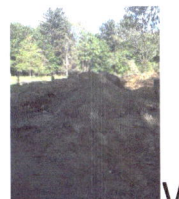What does the soil have to do with our nutrition?

1)

2)

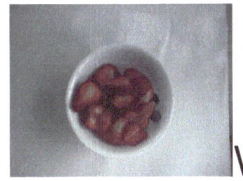Why are probiotics so important?

1)

2)

Tell us something about fiber?

1)

2)

On a separate piece of paper, please write down everything you eat and drink over the next seven days and go over the list with your parents or guardian – repeat as often as they want you to - OK

Notes

Notes